We dedicate this book to all the providers and researchers working to find causes and cures for those impacted by a Lupus diagnosis.

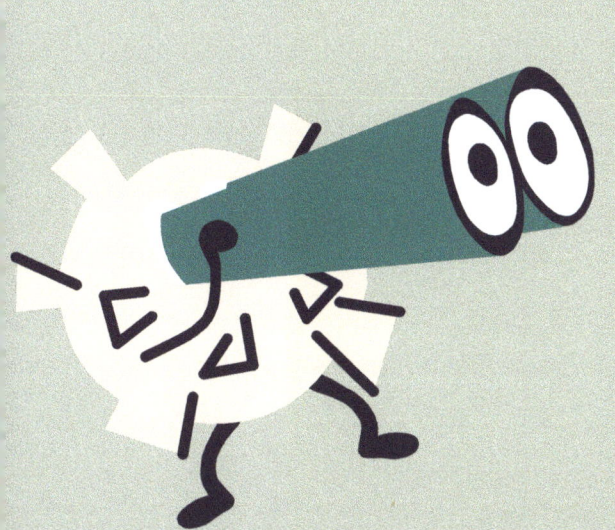
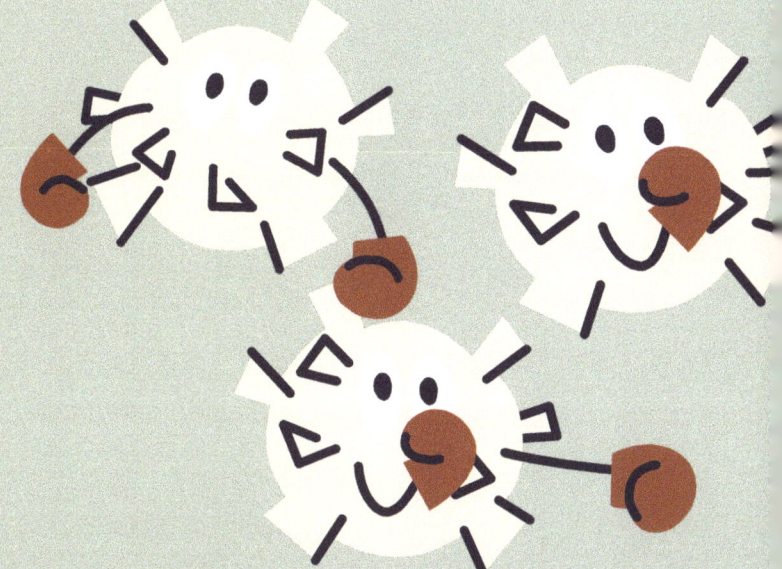

Text copyright © 2024 Child Core Family Support LLC.

All rights reserved.

No part of this book may be reproduced or transmitted in any form or by any means, electronic or mechanical, including photocopying, recording, or by any information storage and retrieval system, without written permission from the publisher.

The only exception is brief quotations for reviews.

For information please contact author at hello@childcorefamilysupport.com

ISBN: 979-8-9987553-2-3

The information in this book is based on our own education, research, and experience. It is designed to be used as a tool to support a child's understanding of the topic of lupus and not in lieu of already existing supports, consults, or medical information provided by Child Life Specialists or other medical professionals.

For more information about Child Life Specialists
and how they can help, go to childcorefamilysupport.com.

Written + Illustrated by Adrienne O'Connor, MS, CCLS
Written by Caitlin McNamara, MS, CCLS, CIMI

Psst... check out pages 42-50 of the book for more information, activities, and tips for caregivers!

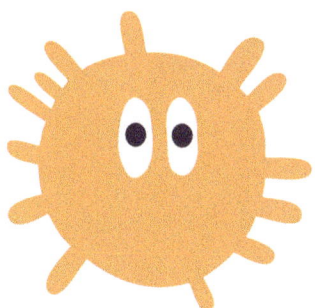

Hey there!
I heard some new words today,
Systemic Lupus Erythematosus...

or

Lupus for short.

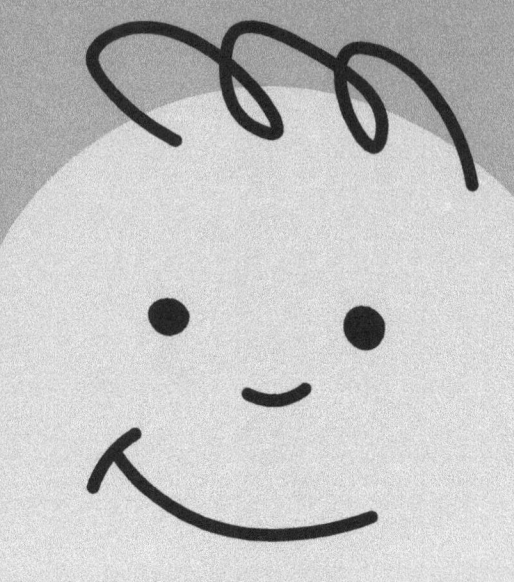

Lupus is something that happens inside the body when someone's immune system gets confused.

Let's learn more by taking a look at how the immune system works.

The inside of our bodies are made up of different systems that all work together.

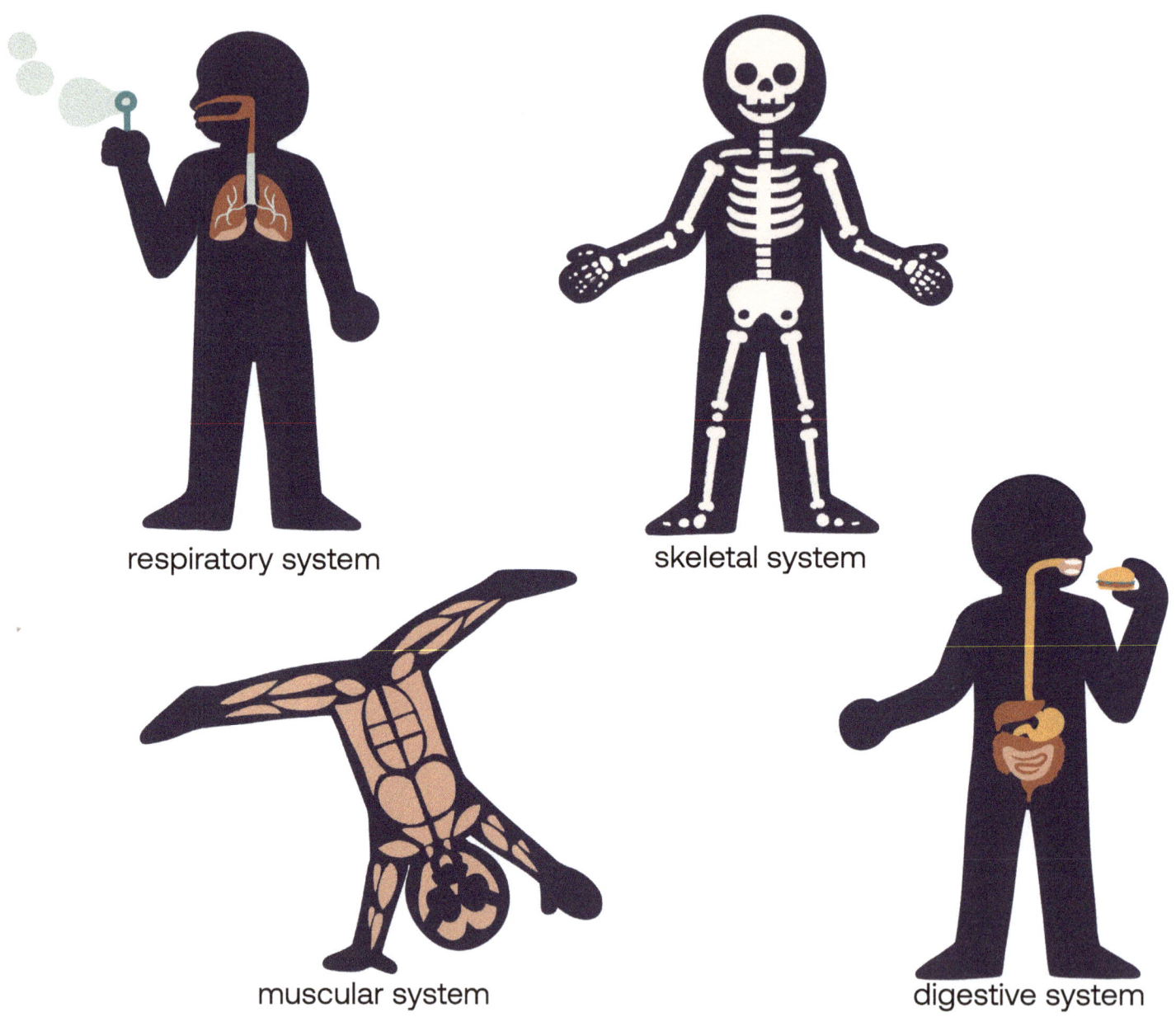

respiratory system

skeletal system

muscular system

digestive system

All of these systems work together so we can be strong, healthy, and do things like

run,
play,
eat,
breathe,
and use our imagination.

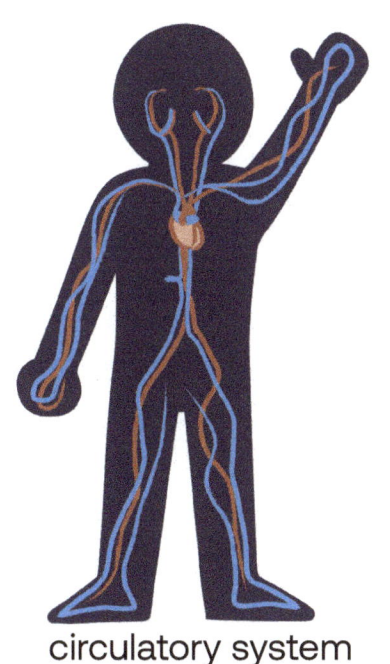
circulatory system

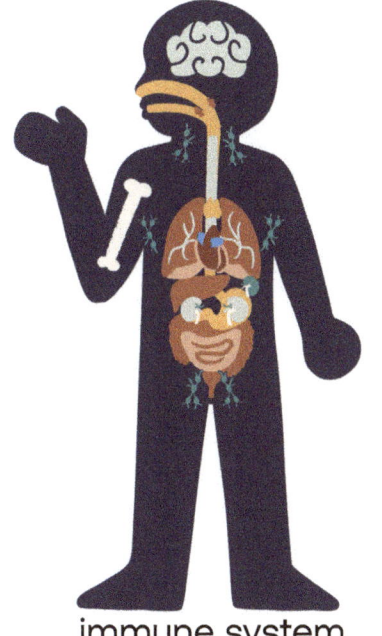
immune system

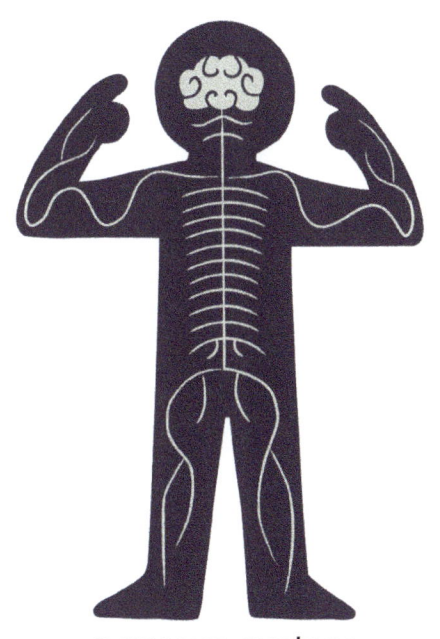
nervous system

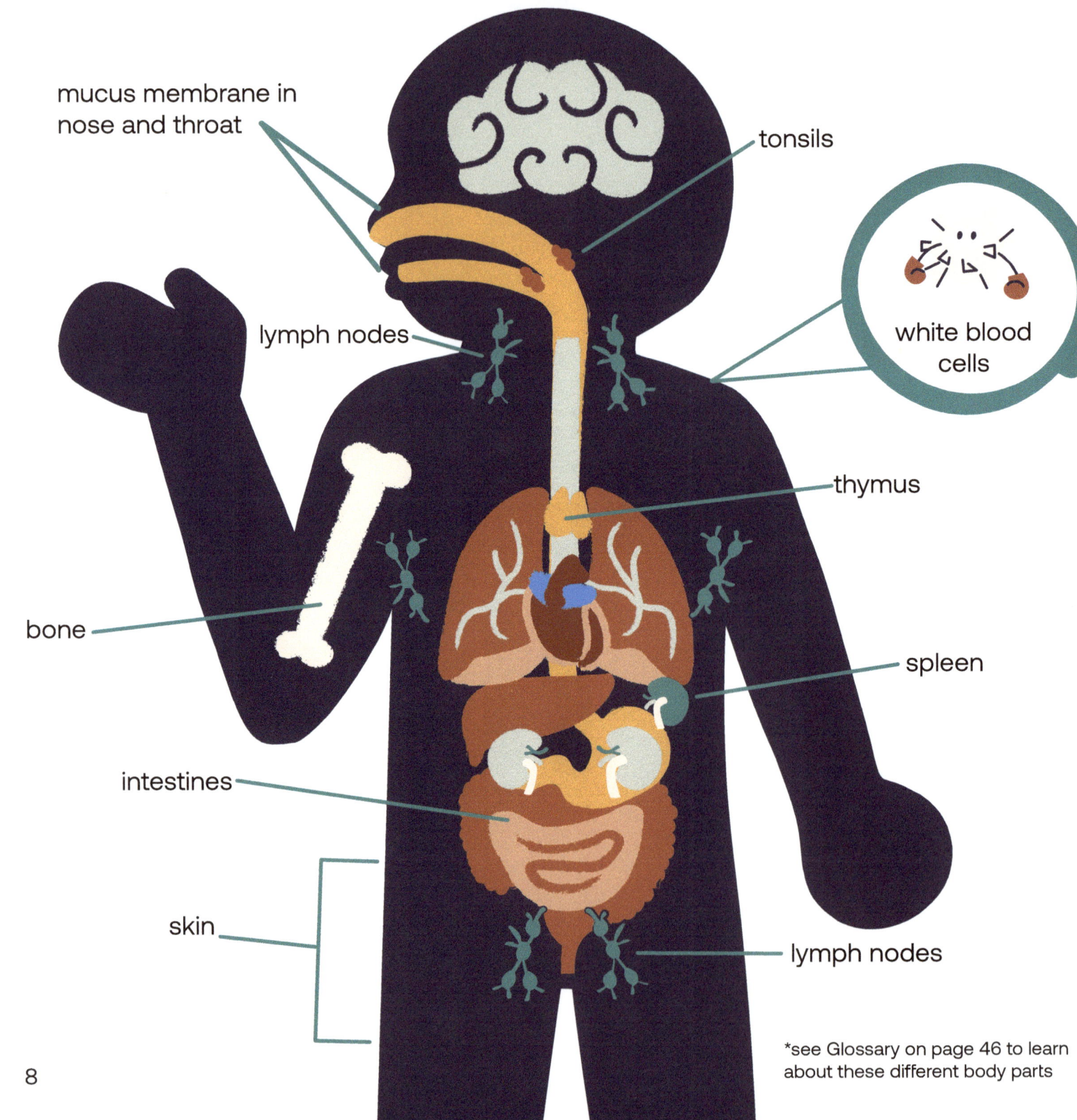

The immune system
is one of these systems!

The immune system is like a team. There are different players that have different jobs, and they work together to protect our body against germs that make us sick. If we do get sick, then the immune system team helps our body to feel better.

Some of the most important team members in our immune system are the...

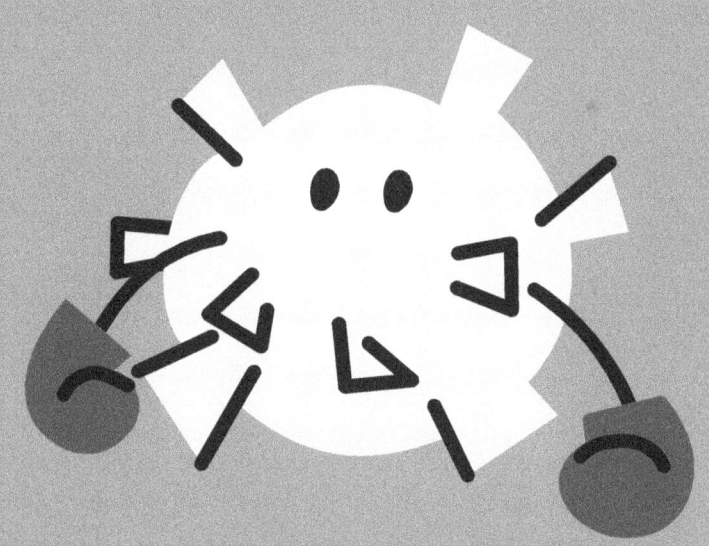

white blood cells.

One of the white blood cell's jobs is to be on alert...

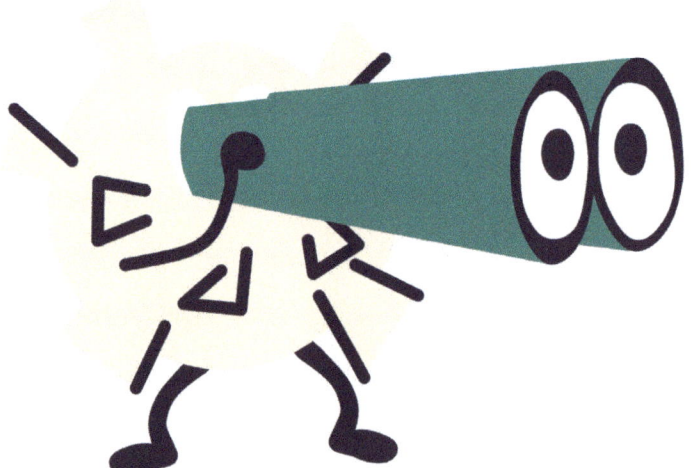

looking for any germs that might have snuck into the body.

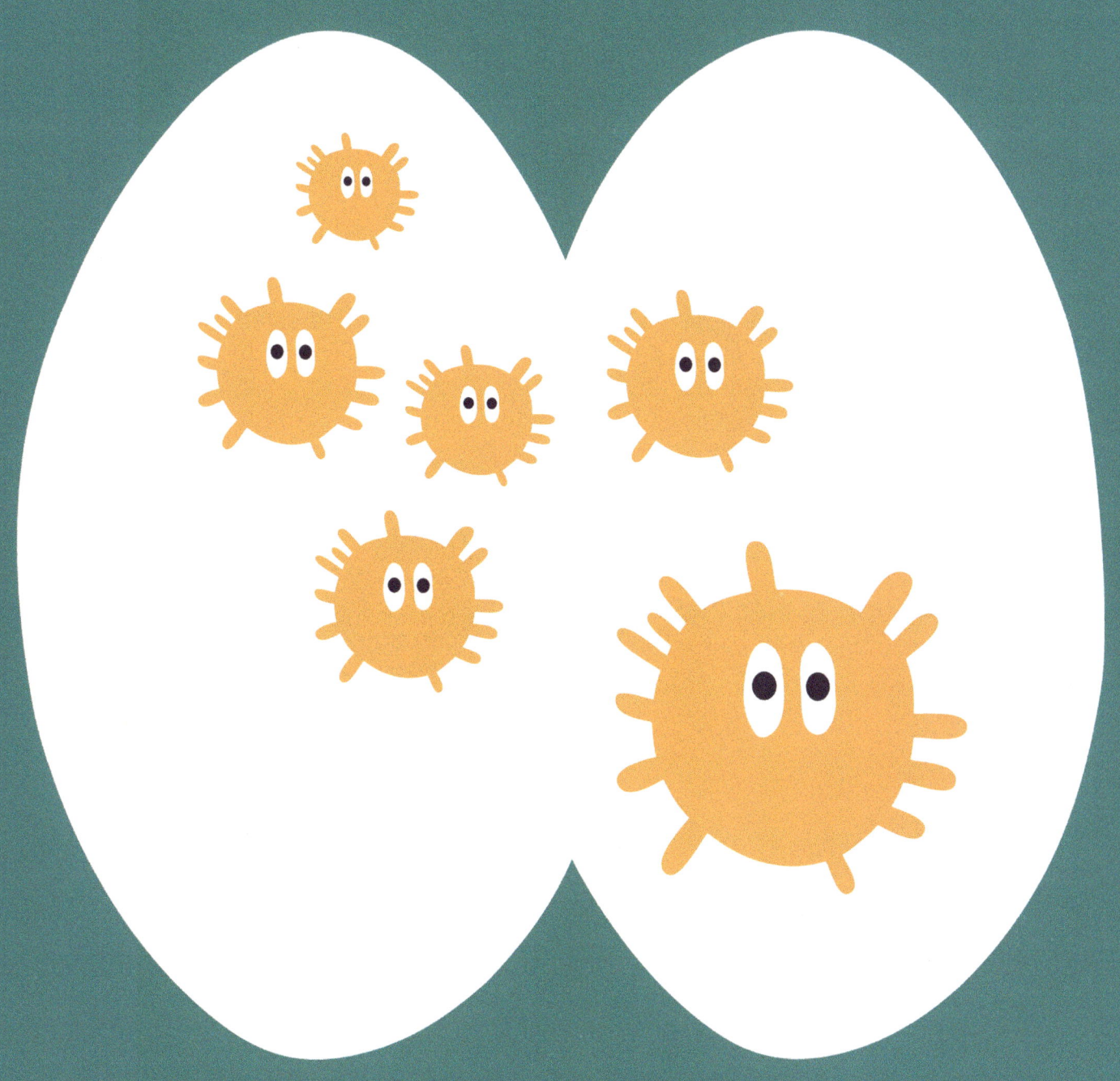

Uh-oh, germs!

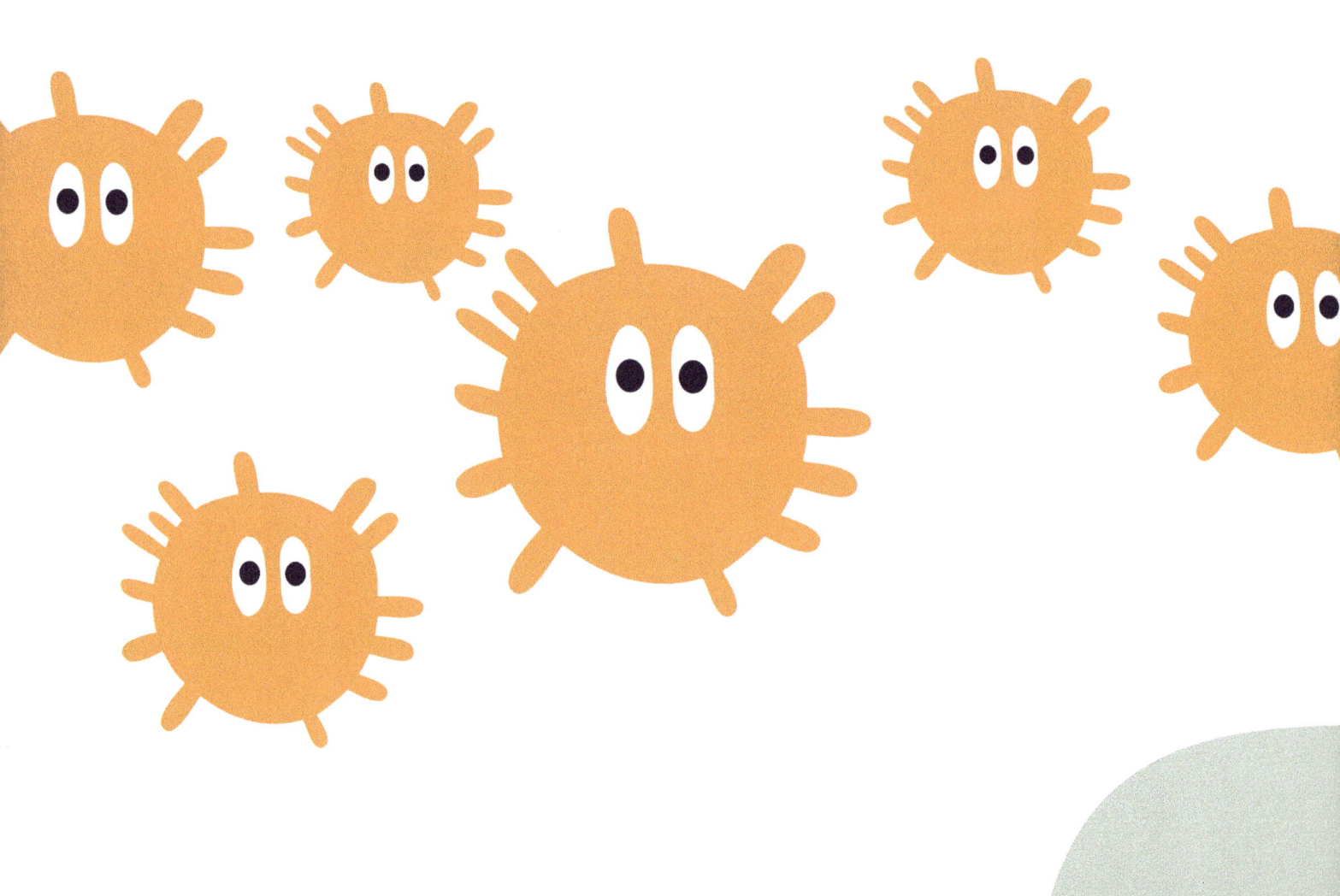

Germs are the tiny, pesky things that live in the world around us, sneak into our bodies, and can make us sick or not feel good.

Once the germ is spotted, the white blood cell sends an alert to the entire white blood cell team...

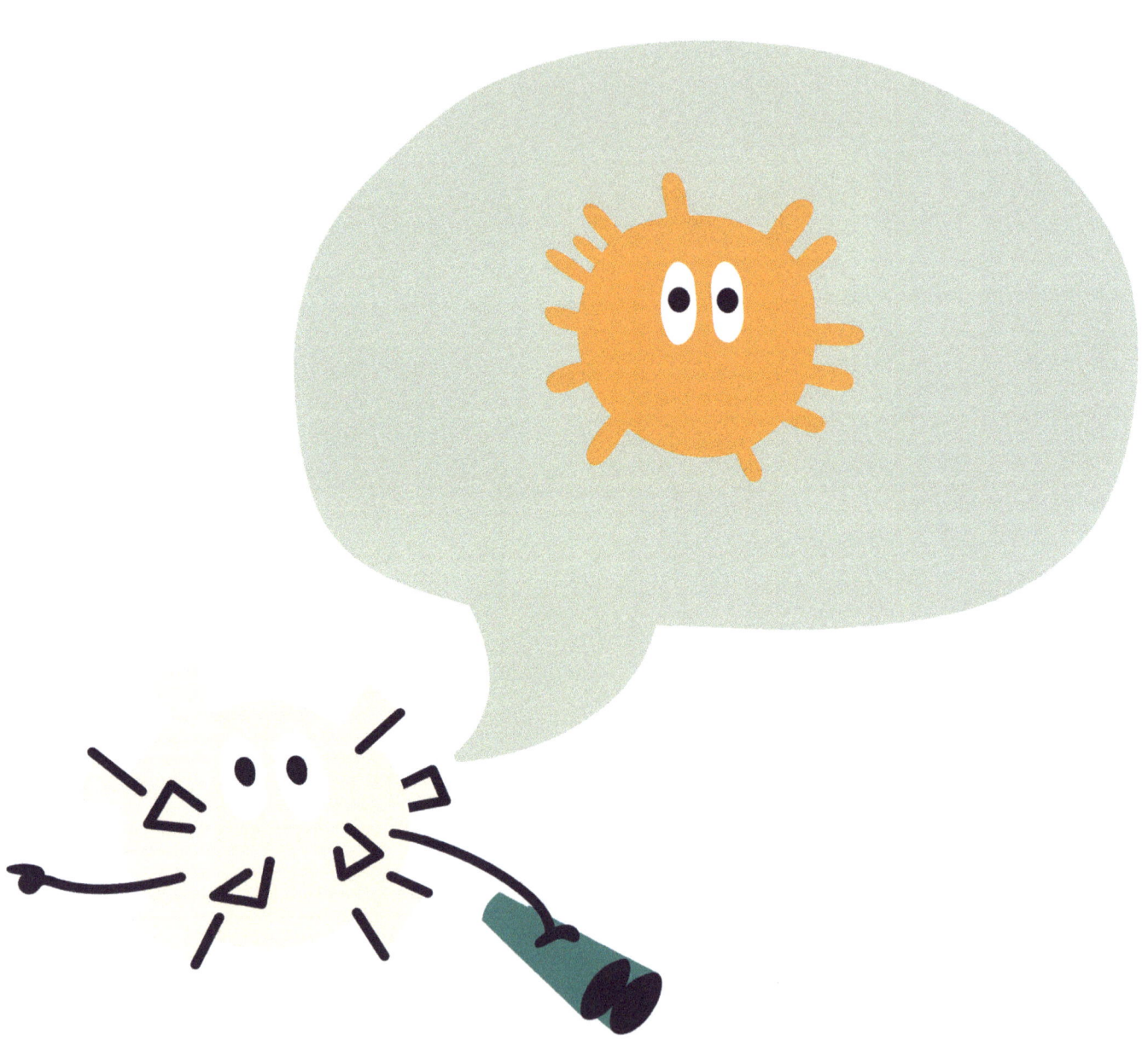

...telling them what to look for and where in the body to go.

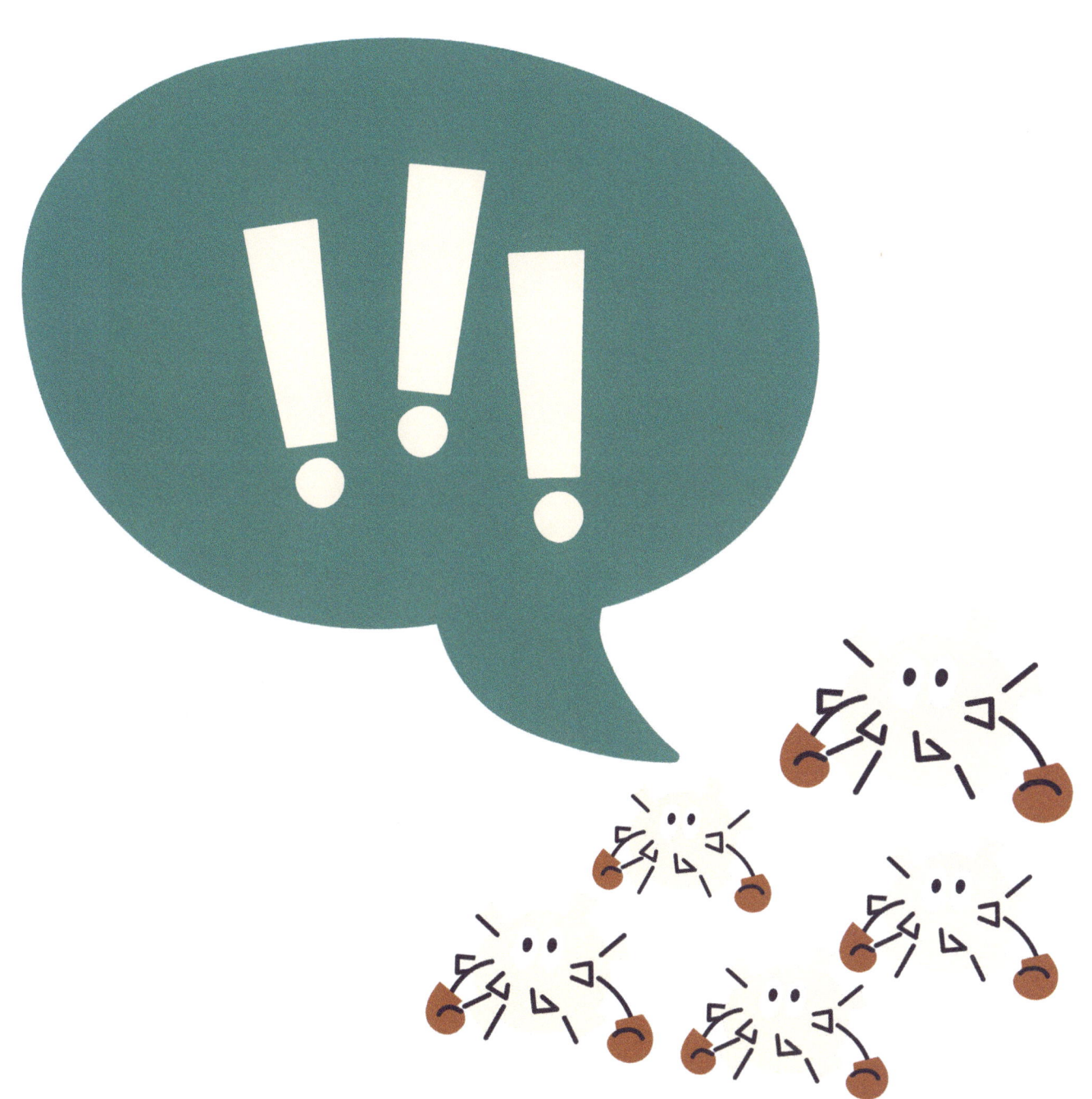

The rest of the white blood cell team is waiting in all different parts of the body for the alert that it is time to jump into action.

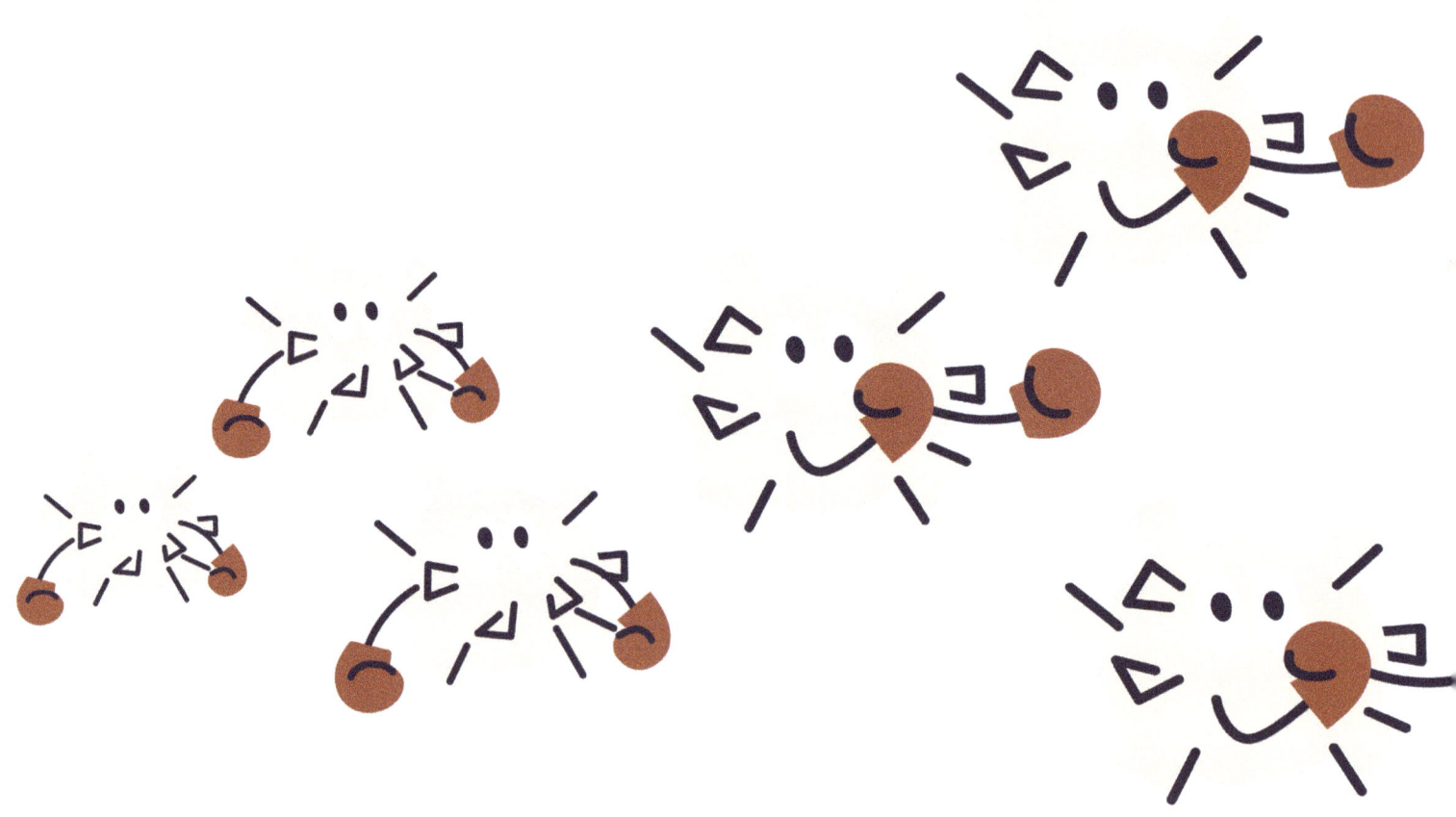

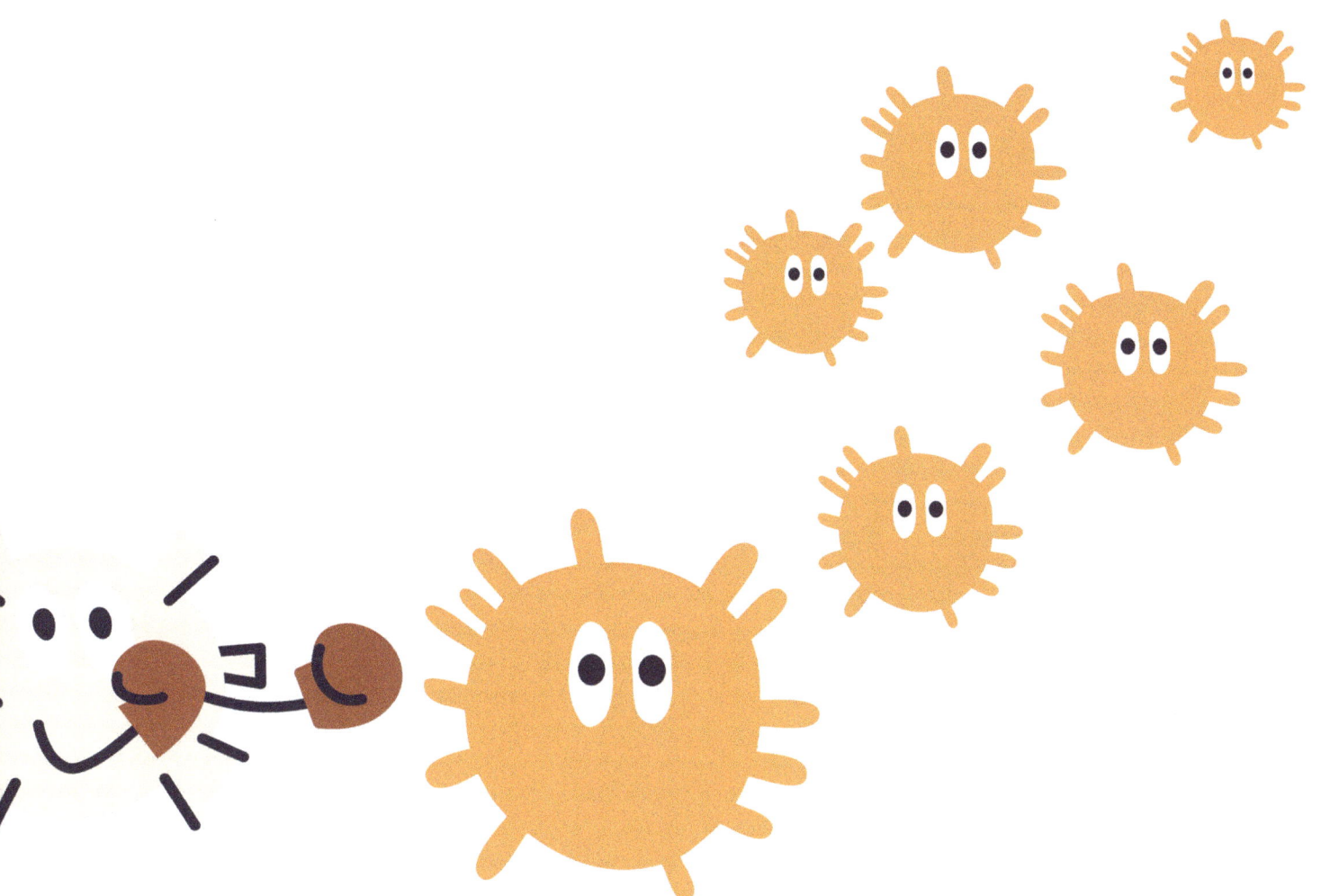

Then, the team of white blood cells join together to fight off the germs.

Our immune system team works really well together.

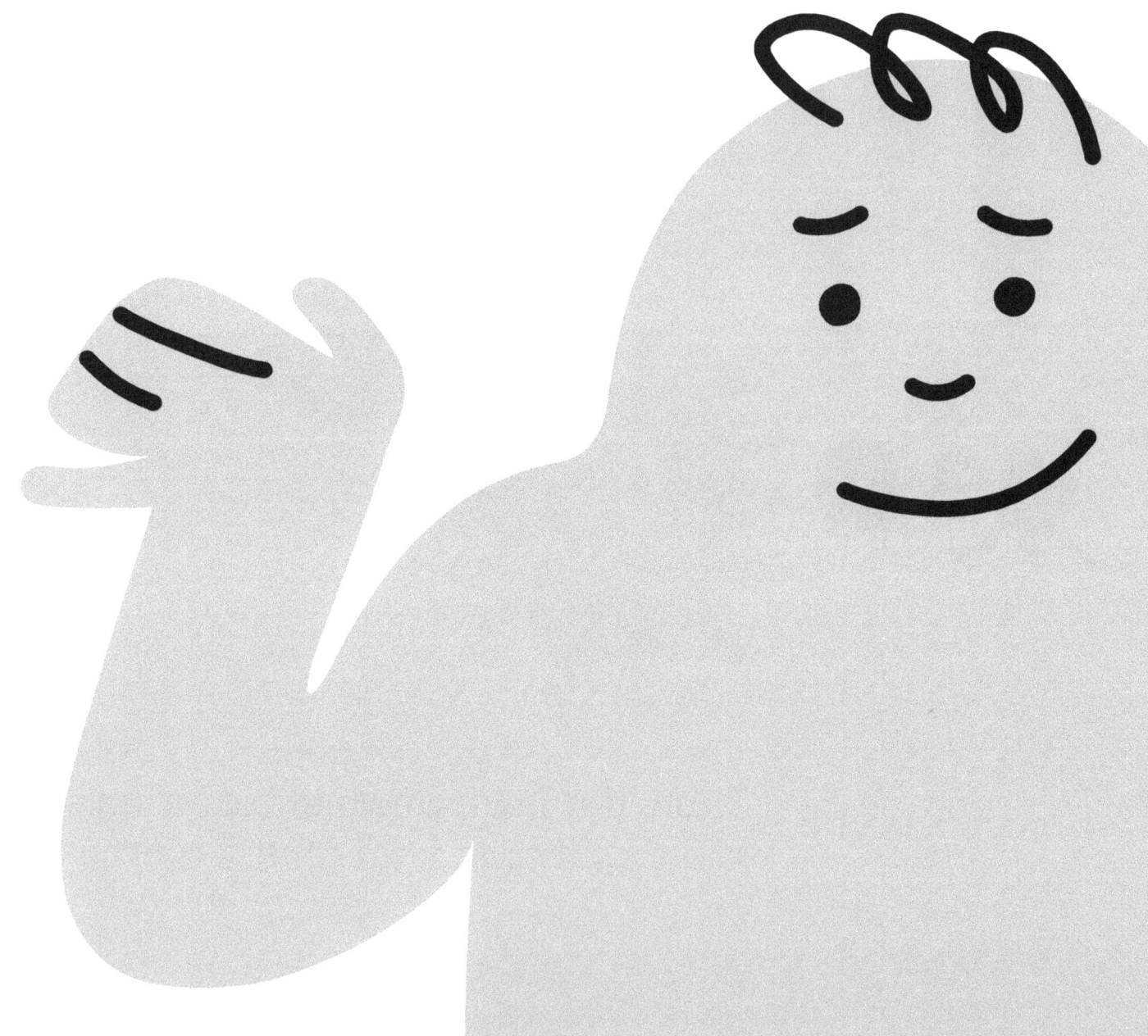

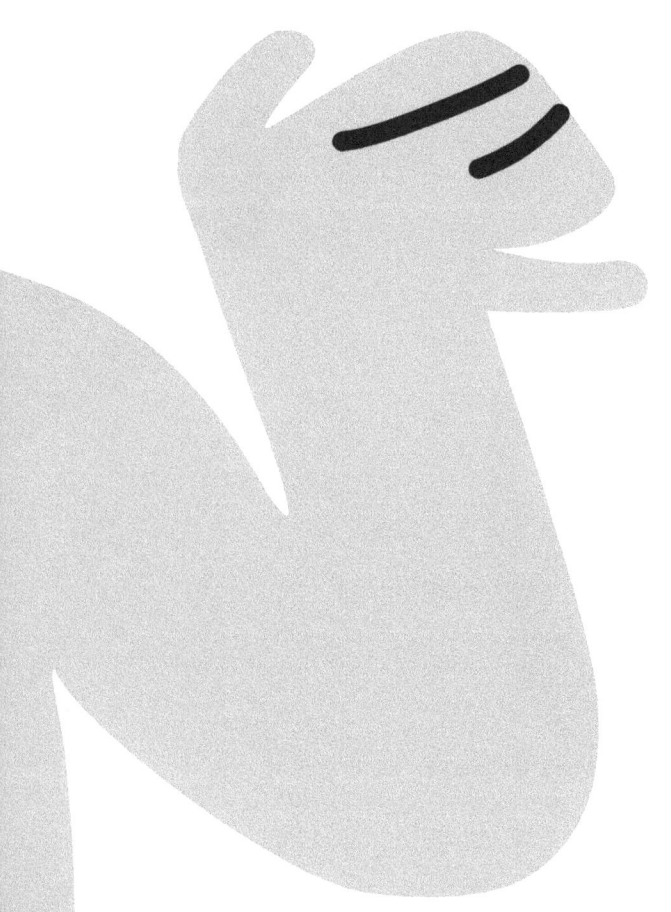

So, what does it mean if someone's immune system gets confused?

Well, fun fact, our entire body is made up of different, healthy cells.

They are so small we can't see them.

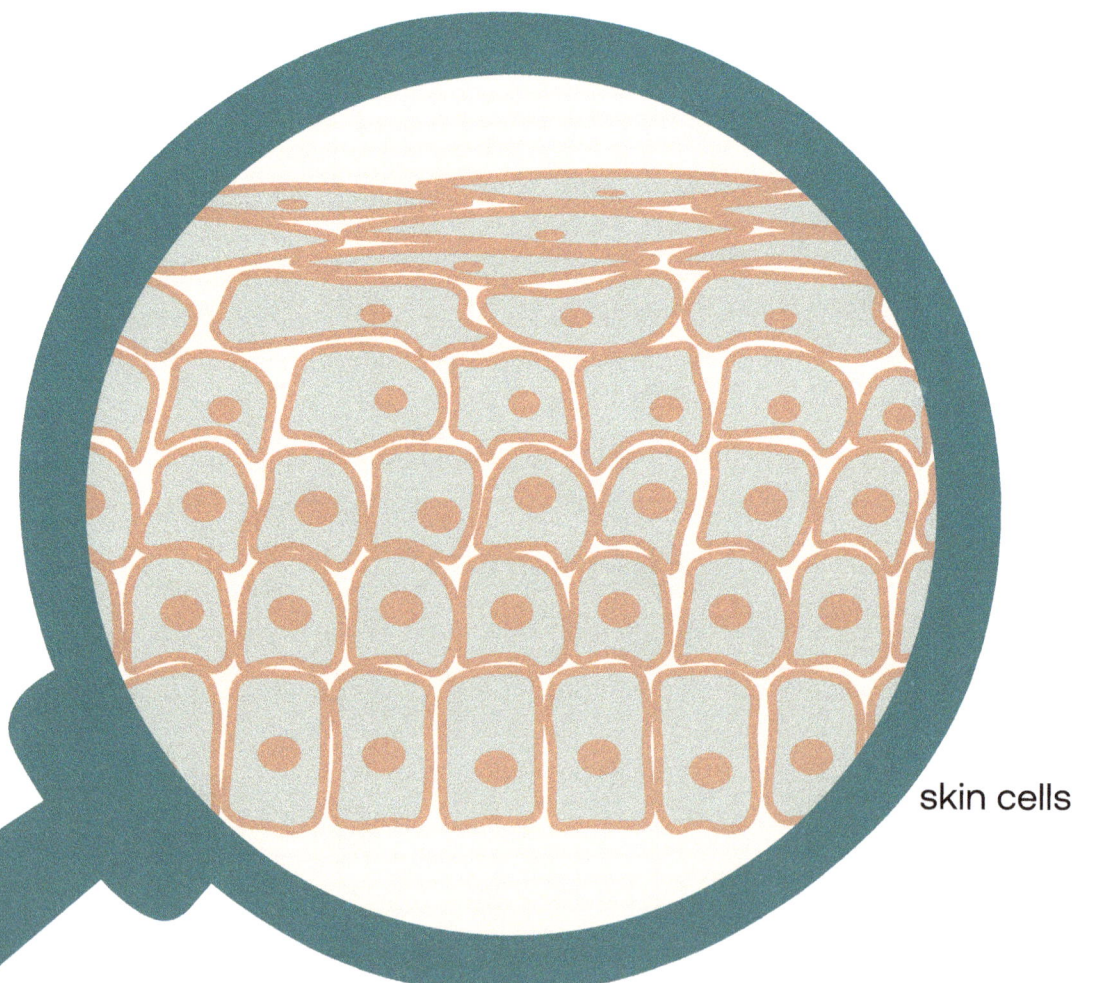

skin cells

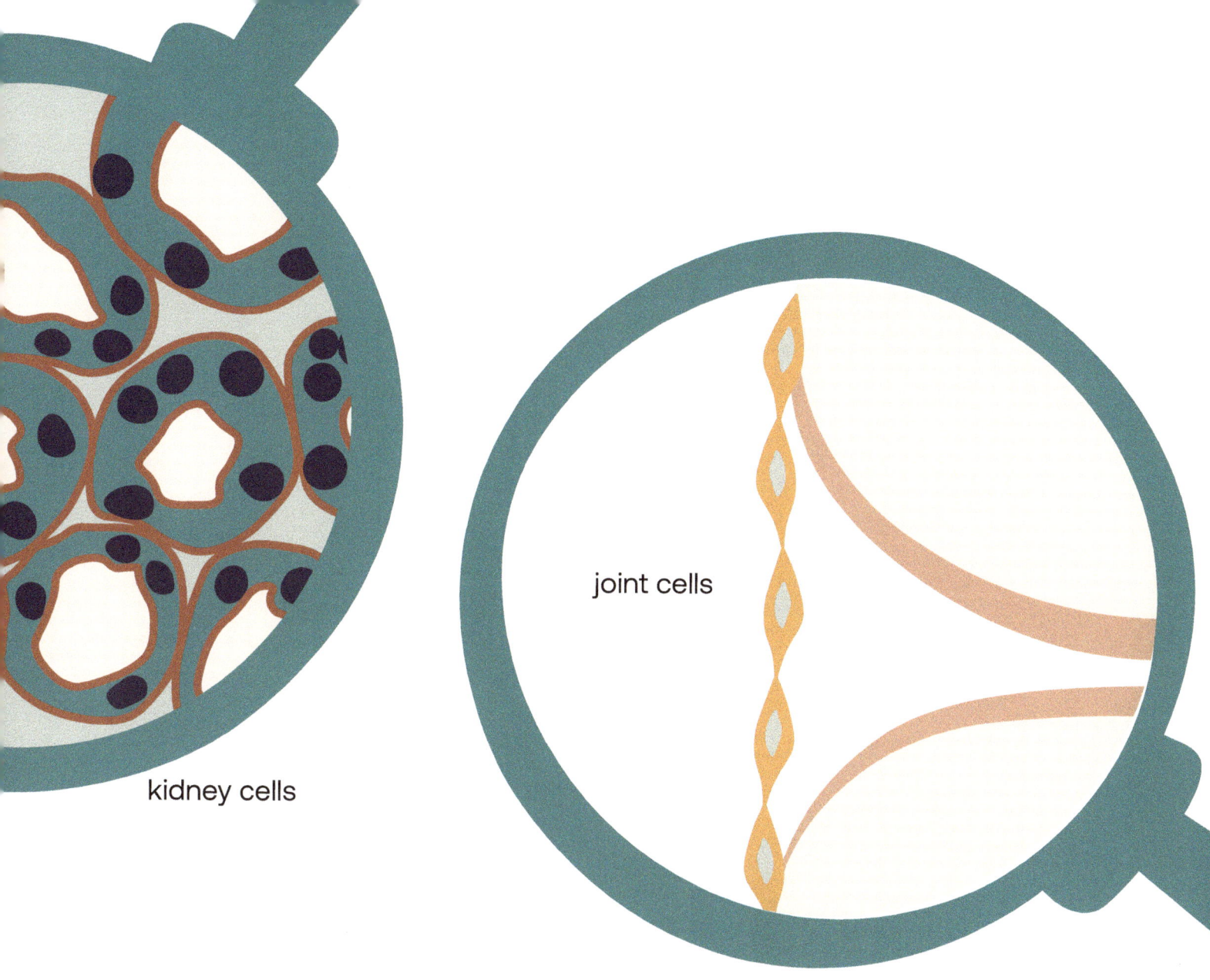

kidney cells

joint cells

The healthy cells make up the insides and outsides of our body.

So, when the immune system gets confused, it starts attacking healthy cells in the body thinking they are similar to germs.

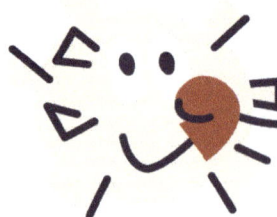

When this happens, it is called an

autoimmune response,

which is different from the healthy immune response that we just talked about.

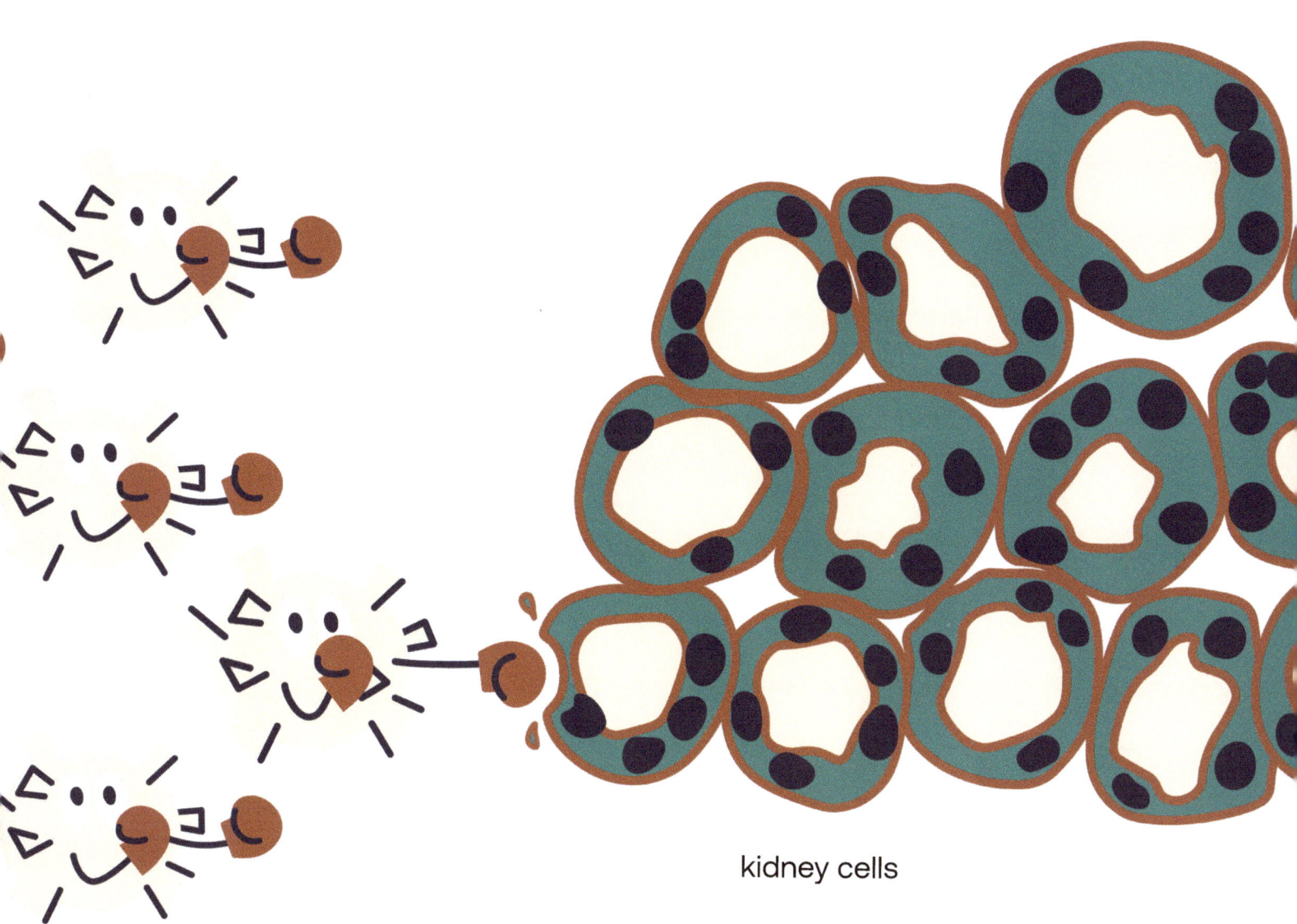

kidney cells

One type of autoimmune response is called

Lupus.

Remember we mentioned that word on the first page?

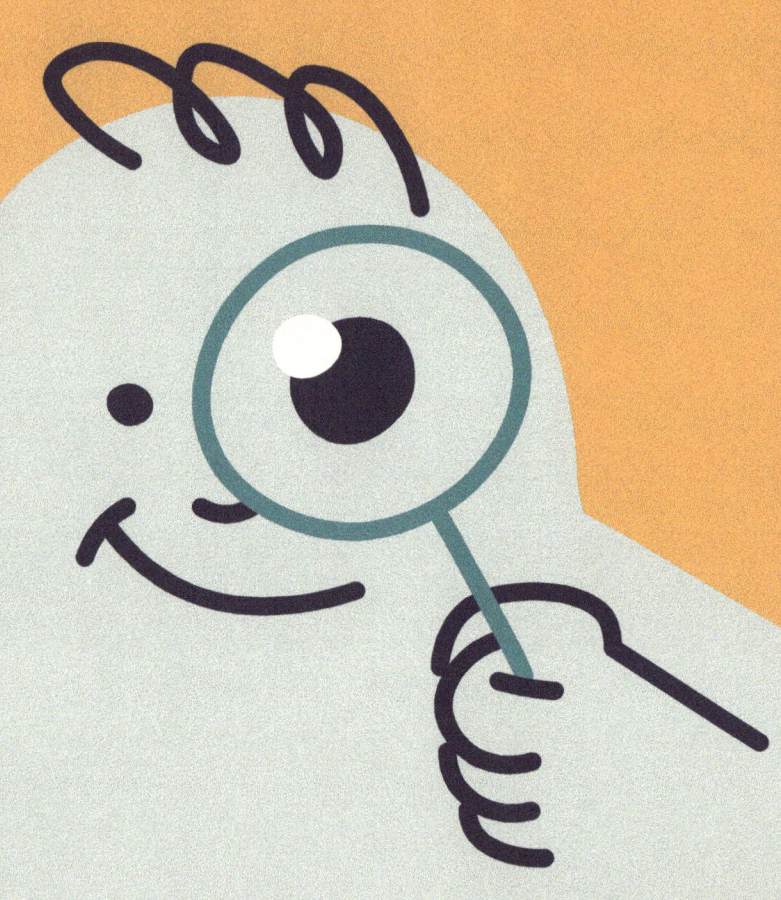

We don't always know why someone's immune system gets confused. It is not something they cause to happen and it is not something they can catch from someone else, like a cold.

Someone can be born with an immune system that is confused, or sometimes it doesn't happen until someone is older.

So, what does it look like when someone has lupus and their immune system attacks their healthy cells?

When the white blood cells attack their own healthy cells, it hurts that part of the body and the body responds to the injury with

inflammation.

To help us understand inflammation think about if someone slams their finger in a door.

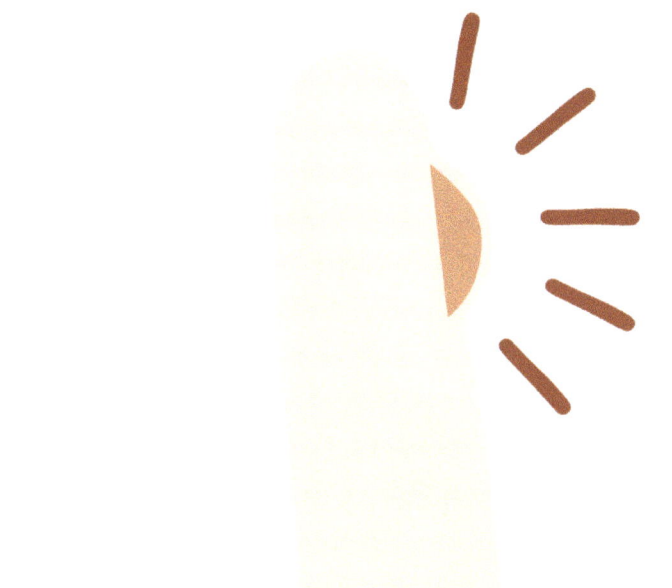

Their finger may feel hot, look red or bruised, or become puffy.

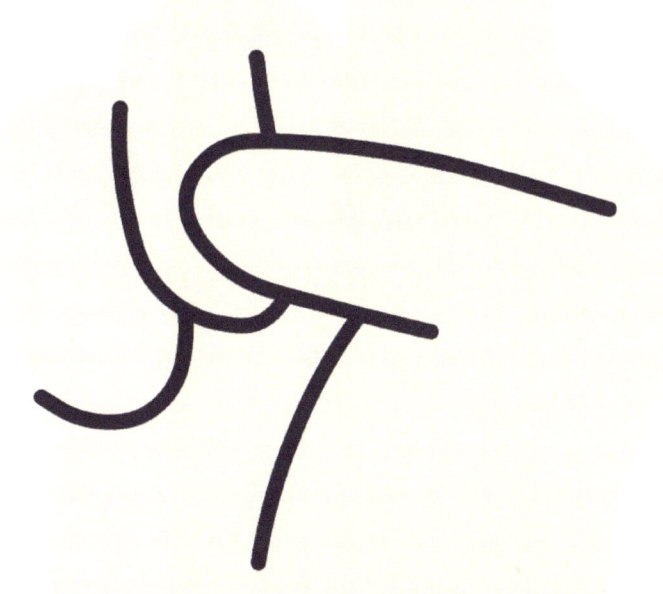

Now, imagine this same thing happening to the healthy cells inside the body when they have been attacked by the white blood cells.

When there is inflammation inside of the body, it can cause different symptoms.

Some symptoms of inflammation can look like this:

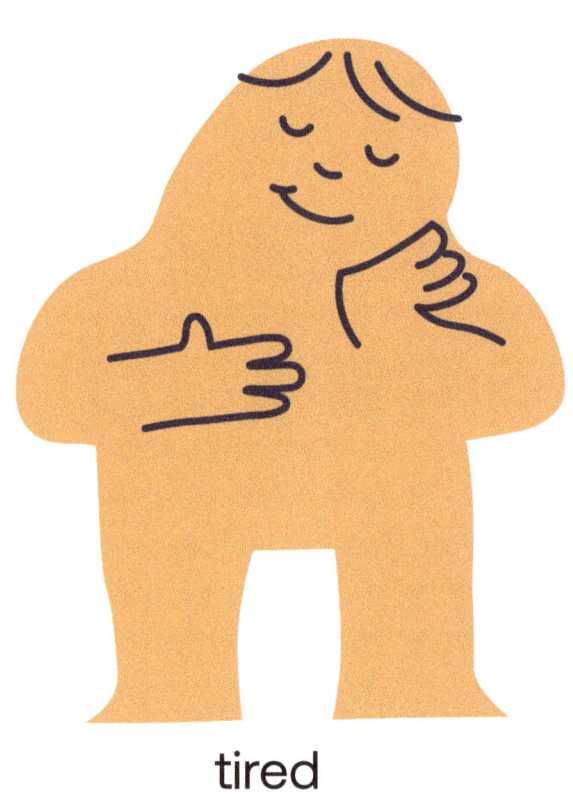
tired

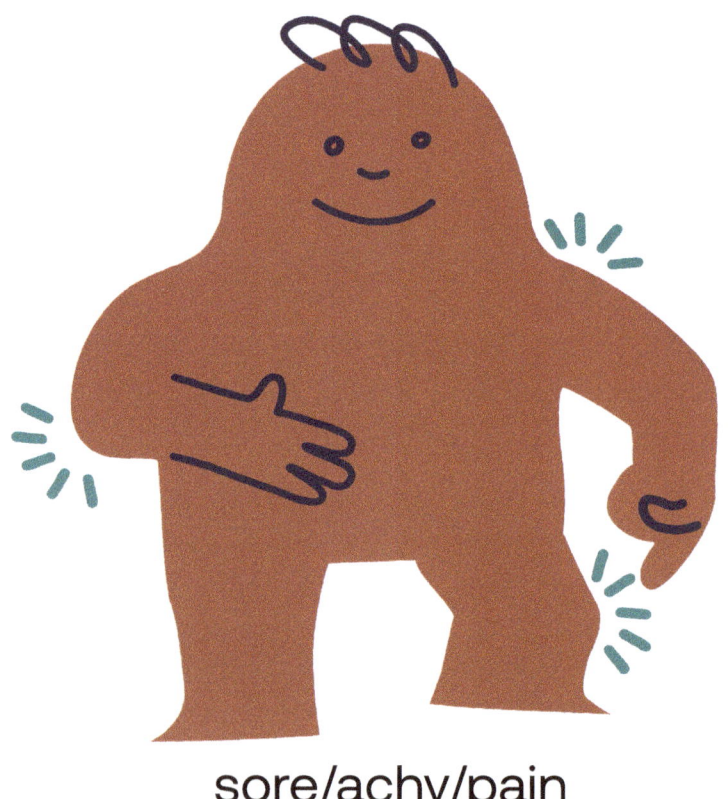
sore/achy/pain

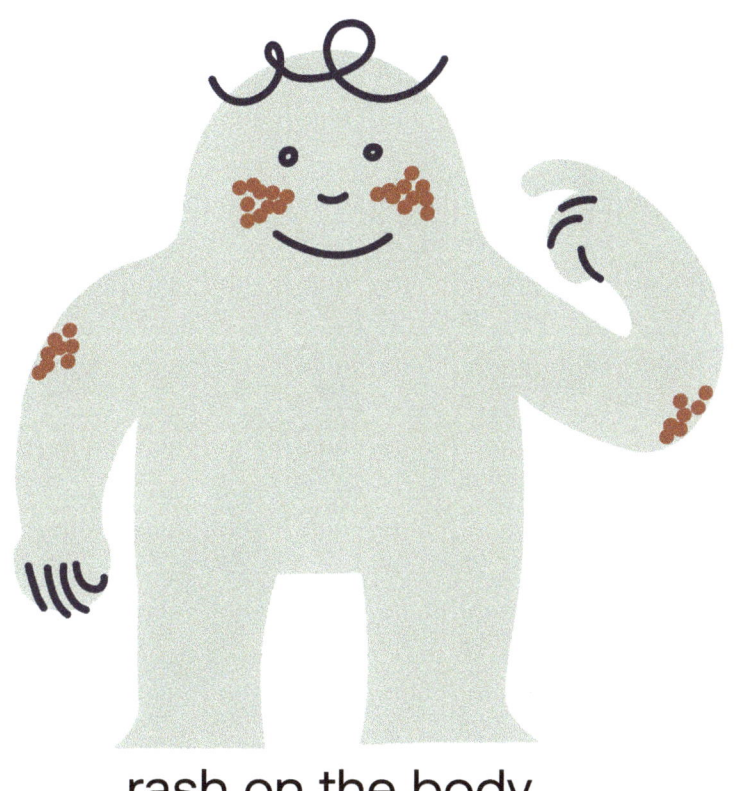

rash on the body

People who have lupus don't always have the same symptoms because the white blood cells may attack different parts of the body.

When someone has lupus they will need to go to the doctor for extra help with their body.

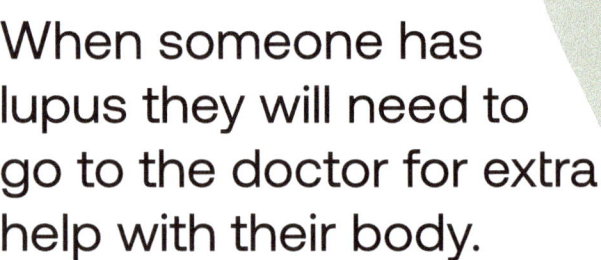

They may need different tests to better understand what body parts are being attacked, or they might need medicine to help with a "flare."

A **flare** is what it is called when someone's symptoms come back or get worse.

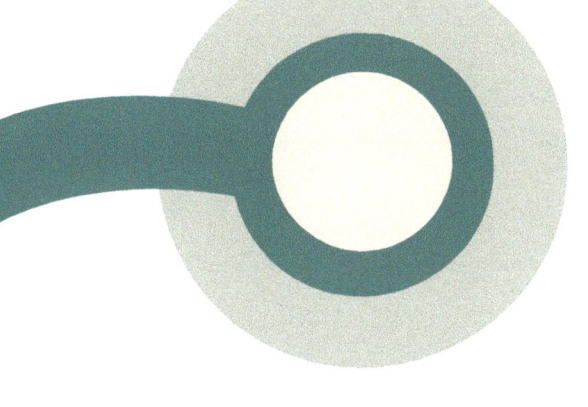

Remember, lupus can cause different symptoms in people, so a medical team will work together to create the best plan for each person.

One way doctors can help someone with lupus, is to give them medicine called steroids.

Steroids helps calm down the confused white blood cells who are attacking the healthy cells.

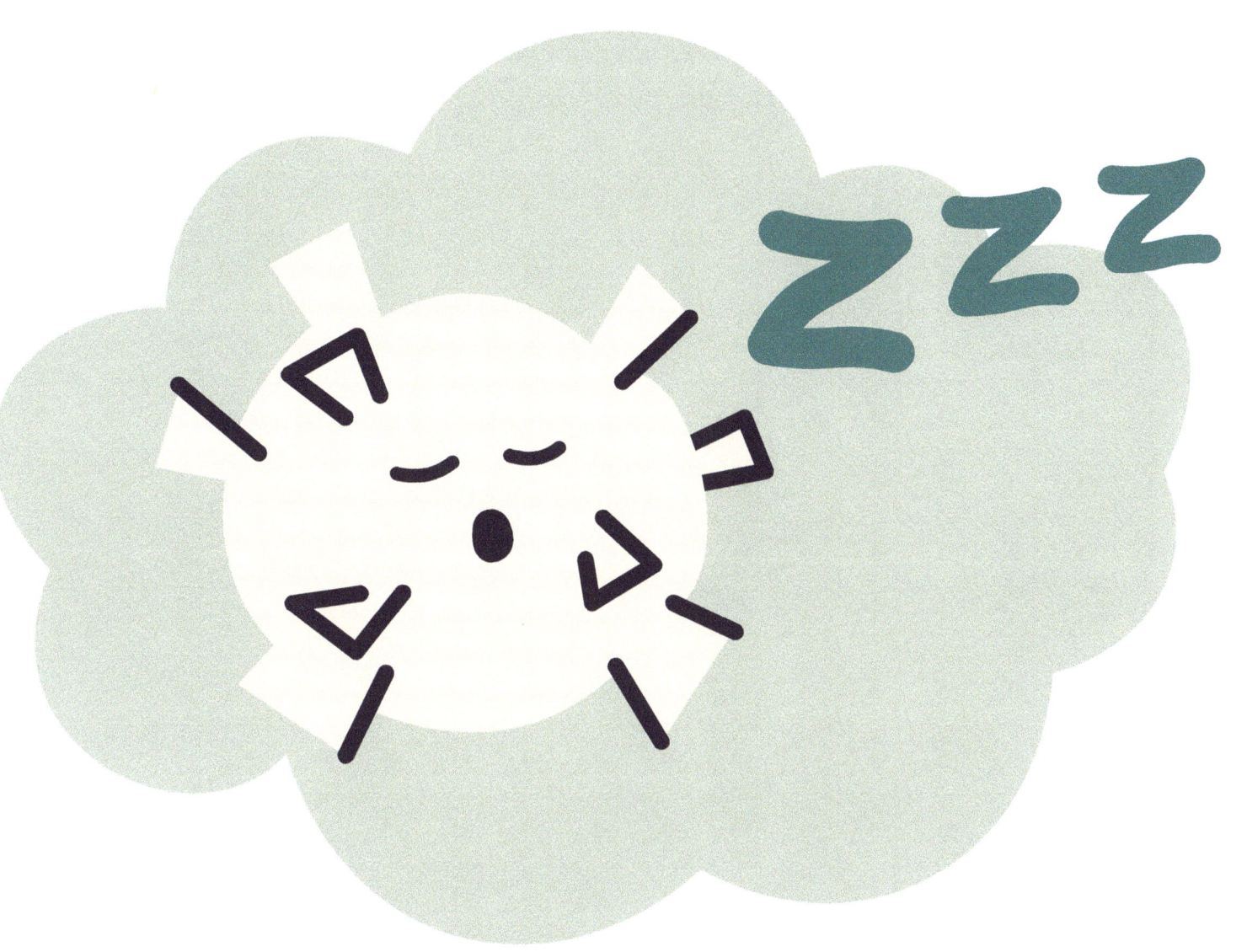

When the white blood cells are slower and more calm, they attack less, giving the body time to heal.

When someone is taking steroids, the medicine targets ALL the white blood cells, even the cells that are protecting the body.

This means that their body may not be able to fight off germs as fast and they can get sick more easily.

So, you may see someone being more careful about germs by

washing their hands a lot,

wearing a mask,

or staying away from large groups of people.

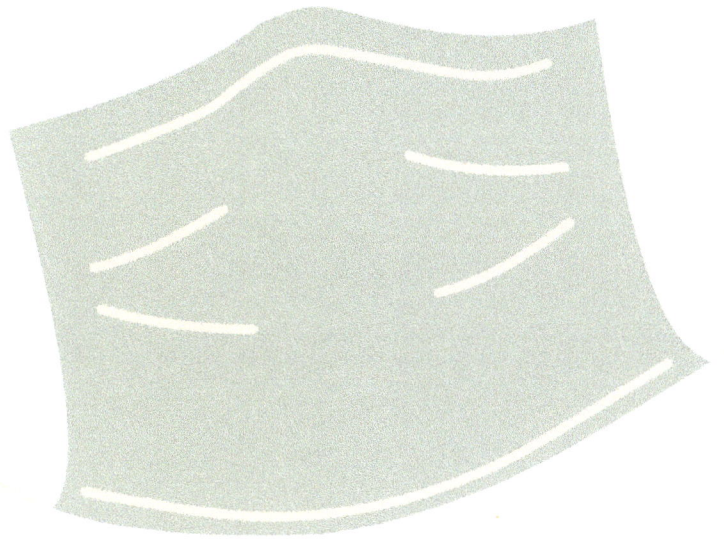

You can help do your part to keep yourself and others safe by always washing your hands, coughing or sneezing into your elbow, and letting grown-ups know if you are not feeling good.

Lupus is known as a chronic condition, meaning that someone will always have it even if they are not having symptoms.

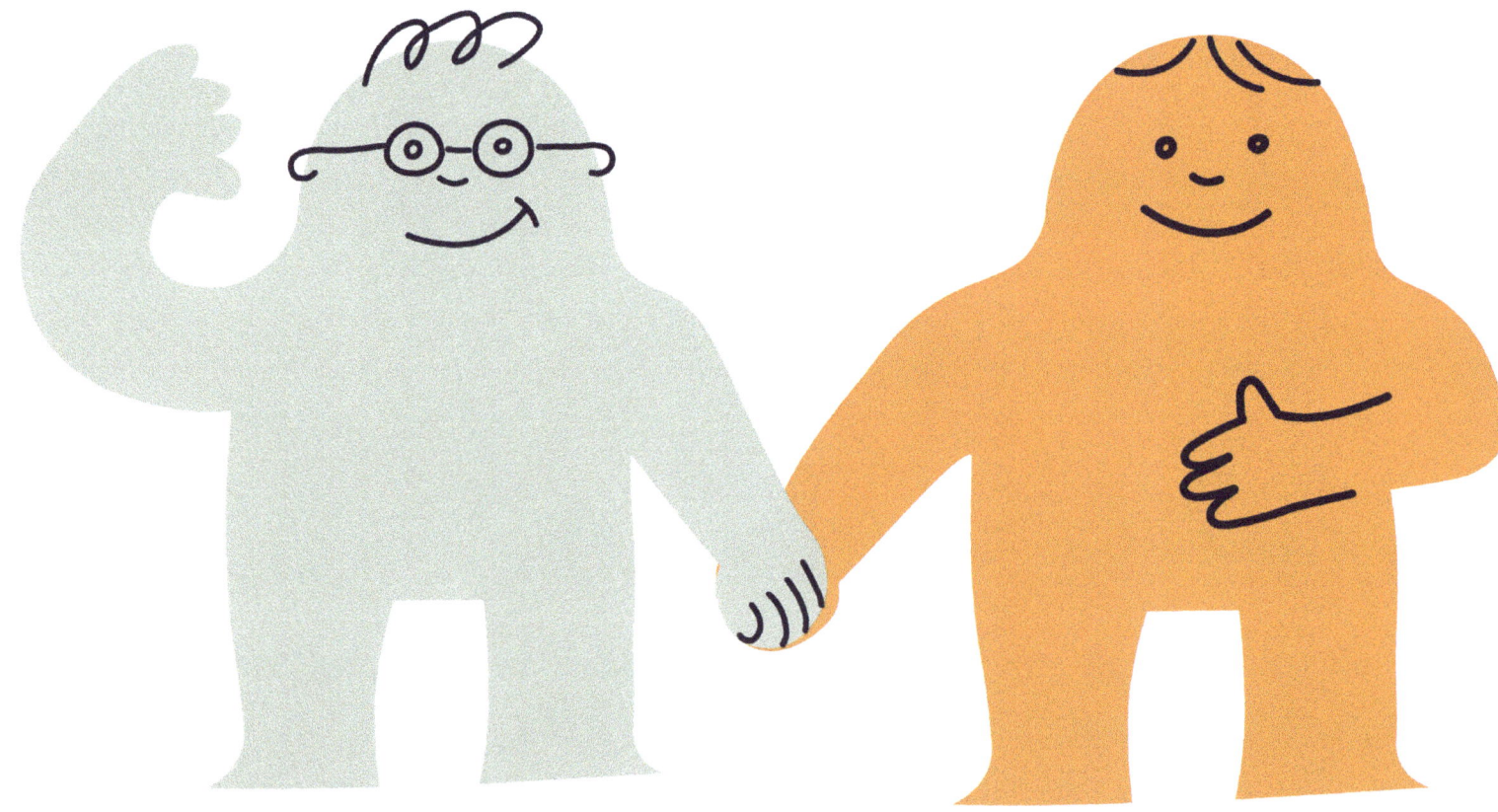

When someone has lupus they can still do a lot of the things that they enjoy doing, such as, eating food they like, playing the same games, going to school, and reading awesome books, like this one!

Wow, we just learned a lot about our immune system and about what happens inside the body when someone has lupus.

It can feel like a lot when learning something new. Sometimes it can be helpful to share with others what you have learned or even read things over again. What helps you when you learn something new?

Glossary

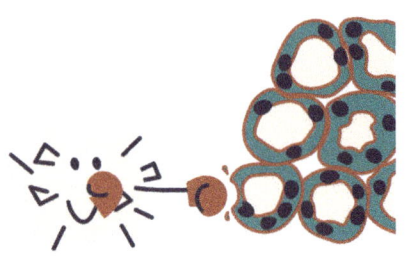

Autoimmune response:

When the body's immune system is confused and attacks its own, healthy cells. Instead of the immune system fighting only germs in the body, the immune system attacks its own, healthy parts of the body. During an autoimmune response, white blood cells travel to certain sites in the body, however, there are no injuries or germs at these sites. Instead of repairing and healing, the white blood cells often end up harming healthy cells of the body. This can cause damage and inflammation to the body's cells, tissues or organs that they attack.

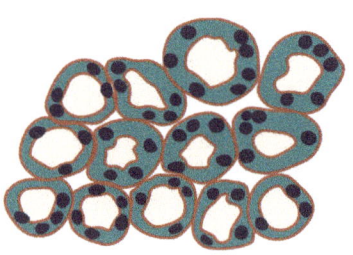

Cells:

Cells are things that make up the body. They are so small you can't see them with your eyes, you need a microscope to see them. Every part of the body is made up of cells, both outside and inside. The body also makes and replaces cells all the time. There are lots of different types of cells and they all have unique jobs that work together to keep the body strong and healthy.

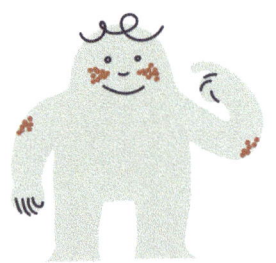

Flare:

When someone is experiencing symptoms or their symptoms get worse, they are having a 'flare."

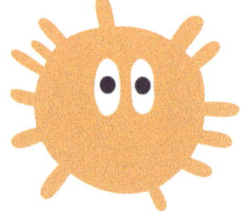

Germs:

Tiny, pesky things that live in the world around us, sneak into our bodies, and can make us sick or not feel good.

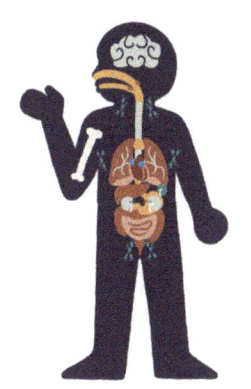

Immune system:

Is one of the systems of the body. It works together as a team; there are different players that have different jobs to protect the body against germs that make us sick. If we do get sick then the immune system team helps our body get better.
Check out the immune system team on the next page

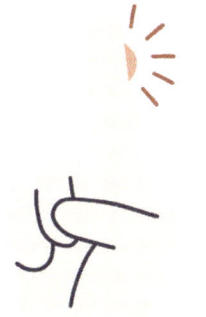

Inflammation:

What happens when the body's immune system, or defense system, responds to germs or injury. White blood cells respond by traveling to the site, which creates more blood flow, and causes those areas of the body to experience symptoms of inflammation; symptoms can include - puffiness, hot/warm feeling, throbbing, or pain. Inflammation can happen inside and outside of the body.

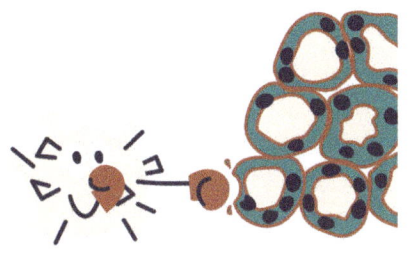

Systemic Lupus Erythematosus or Lupus:

An autoimmune disease that occurs when the body's own immune system is confused and attacks its healthy cells, causing inflammation. The most common body parts involved in lupus include: skin, kidneys, brain, joints, heart, lungs.

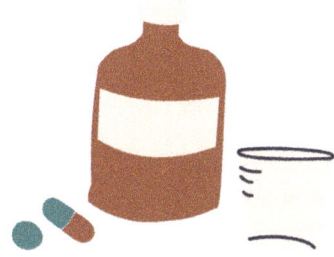

Steroid:

A type of medicine that can be used to help suppress or calm down white blood cells. Steroids make white blood cells slower and unable to attack healthy cells as fast, this leads to less inflammation inside the body and allows the body time to heal.

The Immune System

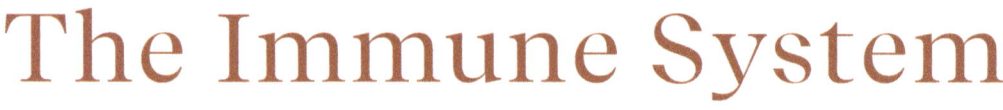

Mucus membrane - Stops germs from getting in the body by trapping them.

Lymph nodes - Where white blood cells are found waiting in the body to get the message to jump into action.

Bone Marrow - The squishy, middle part of the bone is where white blood cells are made and grow up.

Skin - A shield to keep germs out of the body.

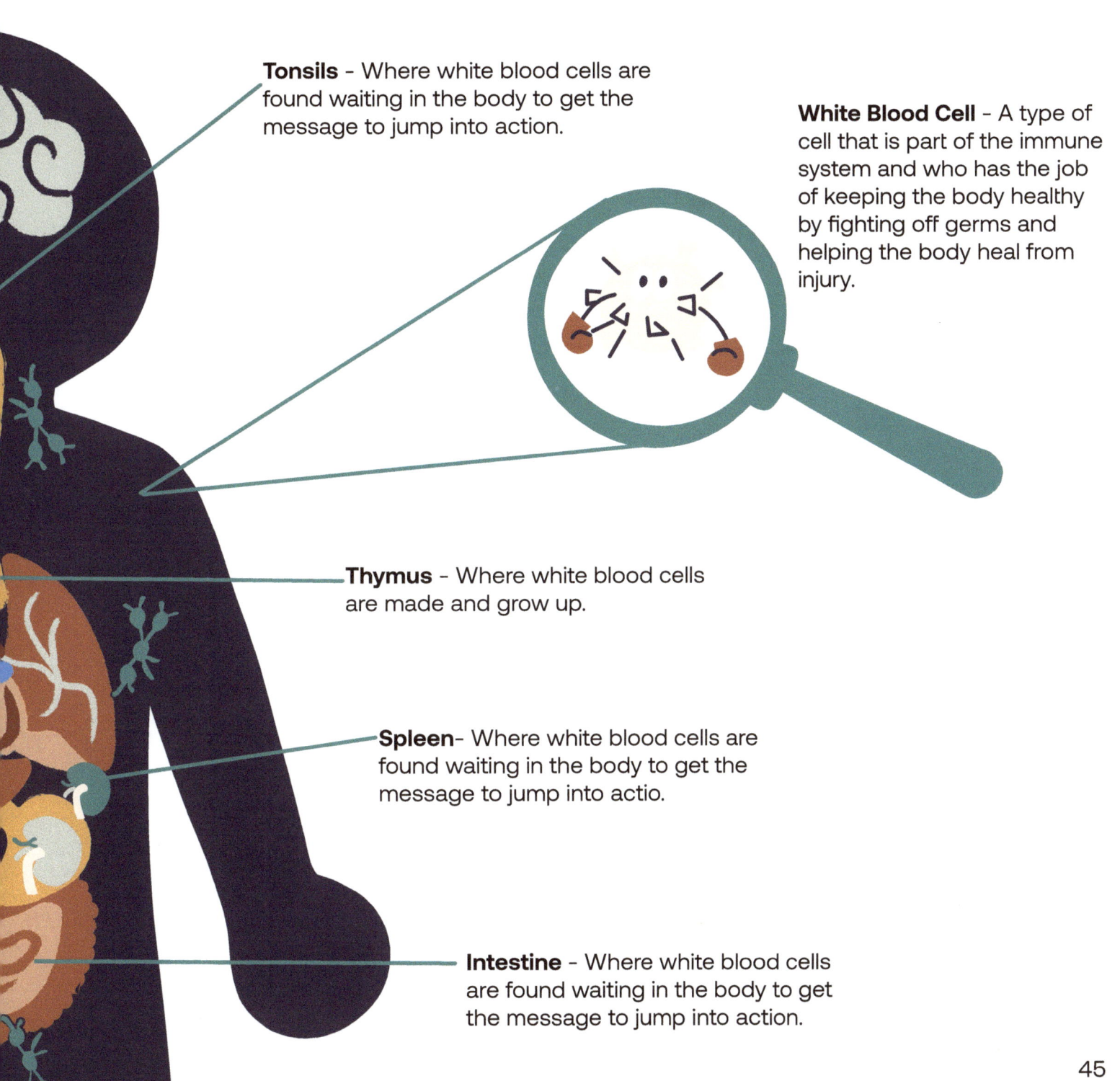

Do you know someone with lupus?

(here is where you can talk about someone you know who is diagnosed with lupus)

If someone was to ask you about lupus,
what would you want them to know?

(here is where you can explore further questions/thoughts or
help your child create their own narrative around lupus)

FOR THE CAREGIVER:
Conversation Tips for Talking to Your Child About Lupus

How to begin to talk to your child about a Lupus diagnosis, for themselves or a loved one/peer.

This book can serve as the entry point into a tough conversation. With this book, you can assess if your child has ever heard these words and if so, what do they understand about them. The learning and understanding process will unfold over time by having different opportunities and avenues to explore these new concepts.

Children understand their world in concrete terms. Identifying physical symptoms they themselves, or someone they know, have experienced or witnessed, helps children make sense of information. For example, if they, or someone they know, have aches/pain and are unable to engage in activities they normally do - work, play - this is a symptom of the white blood cells attacking healthy areas of the body, like the hand joints. Or, if they, or someone they know, are feeling or looking more puffy? This is a symptom they can see that is a result of the white blood cells attacking healthy areas of the body, like the kidneys; making it harder for the kidneys to do one of their jobs, which is to remove fluid from the body.

If you are having a difficult time finding the right words to explain the "why," please contact us at hello@childcorefamilysupport.com to receive some 1:1 support on how to talk to your child about a diagnosis.

Check-in about any questions your child may have or things they are wondering about.

Children are curious about the world around them. It is important to create opportunities for children to have space and feel comfortable asking questions or sharing what they are wondering about. This allows caregivers the chance to clarify any misconceptions (children have amazing imaginations), offer reassurance, and provide information that is specific to the child's actual concerns. This decreases feelings of being overwhelmed with too much information and also focuses on alleviating specifically what the child is worried about.

You may be surprised at the things that are important to your child and thus, what their questions are. Some children need time to process information or they may need time to gather the courage to ask their questions. Therefore, follow up with the child at various times following the book, this communicates to the child that the door is always open to talk and you are a safe person.

How to help involve your child in the medical experience of someone they know who has lupus - friend, loved one, parent, sibling or peer.

When someone is in the hospital or has to go to the doctor's office/clinic frequently or for longer durations, it can be helpful to have activities to focus on. This helps provide an element of distraction, brings a sense of familiarity and comfort, and can facilitate development and healing. Some examples are, have your child color a picture to hang up in a room, create a coping basket with items they enjoy (books, art, puzzles), record a message or video to share, send a lovie item to borrow, or have them be a designated peer helper at school with gathering homework.

Scan the QR code to gain access to additional resources to help guide any adult through helping a child understand and cope with Lupus.

Thank you to all the allies and advocates of the autoimmune communities!

About the Authors

Child Core Family Support is a Child Life Specialist run company that provides consultation, resources, and information to caregivers of children going through medical experiences as well as support for providers who serve these families.

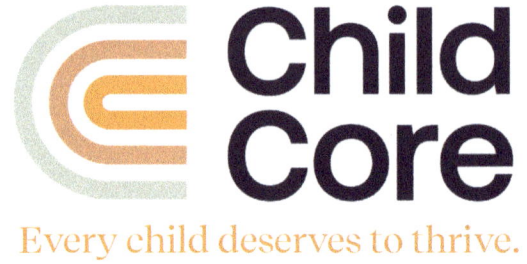

Their educational library strives to equip caregivers and professionals with the tools to feel confident and empowered when supporting a child through medical complexities. Child Core also offers free caregiver guides for talking to a child about a medical experience, and 1:1 coaching to meet the unique needs of individual families.

Find more information, resources, or to learn about child life specialists visit our WEBSITE.

www.ingramcontent.com/pod-product-compliance
Lightning Source LLC
Chambersburg PA
CBHW040004040426
42337CB00033B/5225